All About My Health:
Personal Medical Records Organizer

All About My Health:
Personal Medical Records Organizer

First Edition

Conceptualized, created & edited
by
Kim Clarke

KCLB|P|R|E|S|S

First Edition – July 2014

Published by KCLB | Press
(USA)

Inquiries: kc@kimclarke.info

ISBN-13: 978-0692233849

Cover Photography: © Leelaryonkul/Fotolia
Cover Design: Kim Clarke

In memory of the wonderful caregivers
who paid the ultimate price.

SECTIONS

1 CONTACT INFORMATION

This organizer belongs to --	
Name:	
Cell Phone:	
Phone 2:	
Email:	
Other contact methods:	
This organizer contains information from ___/___/___ through ___/___/___	

This book contains my personal medical information. If found, please safeguard it and contact me using the contact information above. For email, please write "I FOUND YOUR MEDICAL RECORDS BOOK" on the subject line, so I have a better chance of noticing it.

Thank you in advance.

LOCAL HOSPITAL INFORMATION
Keep this information updated!

Nearest hospital (to my residence) --
Hospital Name:

Address (include zip code):

Phone #(s):

****
Other hospitals nearby --
Hospital Name:

Address (include zip code):

Phone #(s):

****
Hospital Name:

Address (include zip code):

Phone #(s):

****

Additional Info:

2 PERSONAL INFORMATION

This information was last updated on: ____/____/20____	
Height	
Weight	
Blood Type	
Ethnicity/Race	
PRIMARY Health Insurance **1. ID/Member #** **2. Policy #** **3. Group #** **4. Effective Date(s)** **5. Employer-sponsored or Self-paid insurance?**	____________________ 1. 2. 3. 4. 5.
Policy Holder's Name	
I am the policy holder's--	Dependent ____ Spouse ____ (check one)

PERSONAL INFORMATION (cont'd)

This information was last updated on: ____/____/20____	
Have secondary health insurance?	Yes____ No____
SECONDARY Health Insur. **1. ID/Member #** **2. Policy #** **3. Group #** **4. Effective Date(s)** **5. Employer-sponsored or Self-paid insurance?**	____________________ 1. 2. 3. 4. 5.
Policy Holder's Name	
I am the policy holder's--	Dependent ____ Spouse ____ (check one)

Member Services Phone # for PRIMARY health insurance:

____

If health insurance is employer-sponsored, provide your (or the policy holder's) employer information:

Name of Company________________________________

Address ______________________________________

____

____

Phone ____

Years Employed -- *from* ____________ *to* ____________

Member Services Phone # for SECONDARY health insurance:

____

If health insurance is employer-sponsored, provide your (or the policy holder's) employer information:

Name of Company______________________________

Address ______________________________________

____

____

Phone ____

Years Employed -- *from* ___________ *to* ____________

COPIES OF HEALTH INSURANCE CARD(S)

Make a copy of the front and back of your current health insurance card(s) and tape here and on the next page, if necessary. Do not permanently affix, so that you can update as needed.

COPIES OF HEALTH INSURANCE CARD(S) – (cont'd)

3 ALLERGIES

Potentially LIFE-THREATENING Allergies
(if none, please check here ____)

☠Allergen:

Date allergy diagnosed:

Symptom(s) of exposure:

What action to take if I am exposed:______________________________

____

____

____

☠Allergen:

Date allergy diagnosed:

Symptom(s) of exposure:

What action to take if I am exposed:______________________________

____

____

____

Potentially LIFE-THREATENING Allergies (cont'd)
(if none, please check here ____)

☠Allergen:

Date allergy diagnosed:

Symptom(s) of exposure:

What action to take if I am exposed:________________________

____

____

____

☠Allergen:

Date allergy diagnosed:

Symptom(s) of exposure:

What action to take if I am exposed:________________________

____

____

____

☠Allergen:

Date allergy diagnosed:

Symptom(s) of exposure:

What action to take if I am exposed:________________________

____

____

____

OTHER ALLERGIES

(if none known, please check here ____)

Allergen:
Date allergy diagnosed and/or noticed:
Symptom(s) experienced:
OTC medications/prescriptions/natural remedies that alleviate the symptoms:

Allergen:
Date allergy diagnosed and/or noticed:
Symptom(s) experienced:
OTC medications/prescriptions/natural remedies that alleviate the symptoms:

Allergen:
Date allergy diagnosed and/or noticed:
Symptom(s) experienced:
OTC medications/prescriptions/natural remedies that alleviate the symptoms:

OTHER ALLERGIES (cont'd)
(if none known, please check here ____)

Allergen:
Date allergy diagnosed and/or noticed:
Symptom(s) experienced:
OTC medications/prescriptions/natural remedies that alleviate the symptoms:

Allergen:
Date allergy diagnosed and/or noticed:
Symptom(s) experienced:
OTC medications/prescriptions/natural remedies that alleviate the symptoms:

Allergen:
Date allergy diagnosed and/or noticed:
Symptom(s) experienced:
OTC medications/prescriptions/natural remedies that alleviate the symptoms:

OTHER ALLERGIES (cont'd)
(if none known, please check here ____)

Allergen:
Date allergy diagnosed and/or noticed:
Symptom(s) experienced:
OTC medications/prescriptions/natural remedies that alleviate the symptoms:

Allergen:
Date allergy diagnosed and/or noticed:
Symptom(s) experienced:
OTC medications/prescriptions/natural remedies that alleviate the symptoms:

Allergen:
Date allergy diagnosed and/or noticed:
Symptom(s) experienced:
OTC medications/prescriptions/natural remedies that alleviate the symptoms:

ALLERGY SYMPTOM RECORDER

Use this page to record symptoms you may develop that appear to be caused by an allergic reaction. Doing so can help you and your doctor pinpoint the allergen.

Date	Symptom	My whereabouts, what I ate that day and/or previous day, used on my skin, etc.

ALLERGY SYMPTOM RECORDER (cont'd)

Use this page to record symptoms you may develop that appear to be caused by an allergic reaction. Doing so can help you and your doctor pinpoint the allergen.

Date	Symptom	My whereabouts, what I ate that day and/or previous day, used on my skin, etc.

Please record your visits to your PCP (primary care provider) and/or allergist due to allergy symptoms on these pages. Detailed information about any prescriptions for allergies should be listed in Section 10 ("Prescriptions")

Date	Doctor	Reason for Visit/Outcome

Please record your visits to your PCP (primary care provider) and/or allergist due to allergy symptoms on these pages. Detailed information about any prescriptions for allergies should be listed in Section 10 ("Prescriptions")

Date	Doctor	Reason for Visit/Outcome

SPECIAL ALLERGY TREATMENTS - If you have received any special treatments for your allergies (immunotherapy a.k.a. "allergy shots", etc.), record them here.

Date	Doctor	Allergy Treatment

NOTES/EXTRA INFORMATION
Re: Allergies

NOTES/EXTRA INFORMATION
Re: Allergies

4 IN CASE OF EMERGENCY

This section was last updated on ____/____/20____

Note: *Local <u>hospital</u> information is on page 2;*
other <u>local emergency assistance</u> #'s are on page 21.

In case of a medical emergency, please contact the following:

NEXT-OF-KIN (Closest Relative) or SPOUSE/PARTNER
Name: **Relation to me:**   **City & US State <u>or</u> City & Country where they reside:**   **Languages Spoken:**
THEIR CONTACT NUMBERS
Cell:
Home:
Work:
Include country calling codes (international call prefixes), if applicable.

See next page for additional contacts!

SECONDARY CONTACTS – in case of a medical emergency (if Next-of-Kin/Spouse/Partner cannot be reached)

#1 - NAME (and Relation To Me)
CONTACT NUMBERS
Cell:
Home:
Work:
LANGUAGES SPOKEN/CITY/COUNTRY OF RESIDENCE

#2 - NAME (and Relation To Me)
CONTACT NUMBERS
Cell:
Home:
Work:
LANGUAGES SPOKEN/CITY/COUNTRY OF RESIDENCE

#3 - NAME (and Relation To Me)
CONTACT NUMBERS
Cell:
Home:
Work:
LANGUAGES SPOKEN/CITY/COUNTRY OF RESIDENCE

LOCAL EMERGENCY NUMBERS

CONTACTS	PHONE #
Emergency (life-threatening)	911
Poison Control	________________
Police Department	________________
Fire Department	________________
Next-door Neighbor Name:	________________
Next-door Neighbor Name:	________________
	________________
	________________
	________________

NOTES/EXTRA INFORMATION
Re: Emergencies

5 HEALTH PROXY INFORMATION

If you have a **Medical Advance Directive a.k.a. Health Care Proxy a.k.a. Living Will** indicating your wishes in the event you are incapable of making your own medical decisions, please indicate here where the signed document can be located (the document is very detailed and usually several pages long):

____

____

____

____

____

The aforementioned document would include the name(s) of a PRIMARY person (and sometimes SECONDARY person) that would act as your **health care agent** and make medical decisions on your behalf, if necessary. Health care agents need to be provided with a signed & dated copy of the Advance Directive document! You can also have your doctors keep a copy in their files.

Please list the name(s) of your HEALTH CARE AGENT(S) here, even if they are already listed as one of your emergency contacts.

My Health Care Agent(s) is/are:

Name:

Relation:

Contact Number(s):

Has a copy of my Advance Directive: YES NO *(circle one)*

Name:

Relation:

Contact Number(s):

Has a copy of my Advance Directive: YES NO *(circle one)*

NOTE: Each U.S. state has created their own legally-binding Advance Directive/Health Care Proxy/Living Will document. They can be easily found online and downloaded or printed. Do a search for "advance directive" (including your state's name) and you should find several sources. They are also readily available at all U.S. hospitals.

6 FAMILY MEDICAL HISTORY

Relative	Living? Y/N	Age at Death	Cause of Death
Biological Mother			
Biological Father			
Maternal Grandmother			
Maternal Grandfather			
Paternal Grandmother			
Paternal Grandfather			

MEDICAL HISTORY OF IMMEDIATE FAMILY

(information for extended family starts on page 29)

Relative	Known Diseases, Chronic Illnesses, Conditions
Mother	
Father	
Maternal Grandmother	
Maternal Grandfather	
Paternal Grandmother	
Paternal Grandfather	

Additional relatives on next page…

MEDICAL HISTORY OF IMMEDIATE FAMILY (cont'd)

Please list information about the following blood relatives:

Your Siblings & Your Children

Also include the medical history of any **long-term Spouses/Partners** that you have lived with for an extended amount of time. For deceased relatives, include age of death and cause.

Relative	Diseases, Chronic Illnesses, Conditions

MEDICAL HISTORY OF IMMEDIATE FAMILY (cont'd)

Your Siblings & Your Children

Also Long-term, Live-in Spouse/Partner

Relative	Diseases, Chronic Illnesses, Conditions

Degrees of Relationship

First-degree relatives	Parents, children, full-siblings
Second-degree relatives	Grandparents, aunts and uncles, nieces and nephews, grandchildren, half-siblings
Third-degree relatives	First cousin, great-grandparent or great-grandchild

MEDICAL HISTORY OF EXTENDED FAMILY

Medical diseases, abnormalities, serious/chronic conditions and recurrent illnesses among blood relatives.

List any known information for second-degree relatives (not accounted for on previous pages) and third-degree relatives:

Condition(s)	Is it hereditary? Y / N / DK	Relative Affected	Maternal or Paternal side?

MEDICAL HISTORY OF EXTENDED FAMILY (cont'd)

Condition(s)	Is it hereditary? Y / N / DK	Relative Affected	Maternal or Paternal side?

NOTES/EXTRA INFORMATION
Re: Family Medical History

NOTES/EXTRA INFORMATION
Re: Family Medical History

7 MY MEDICAL HISTORY

(For ALLERGY INFORMATION, see Section 3)

IMMUNIZATIONS/VACCINATION RECORDS

You should keep your official immunization record(s)/card(s) in a safe place. They may be required for certain employment, travel abroad and for school registrations. The official records/cards are signed and dated by the medical professionals who administer the vaccinations.

For more information about locating official immunizations records, go to this Centers for Disease Control and Prevention website link: http://www.cdc.gov/vaccines/adults/vaccination-records.html

Go to this Immunization Action Coalition weblink to print out an official immunization record form that you can have medical providers fill out each time you receive a vaccination: http://www.immunize.org/catg.d/p2023.pdf

Vaccines Routinely Administered in the United States

- Hepatitis B (HepB)
- Rotavirus
- Diphtheria, pertussis, and tetanus
- Haemophilus influenzae type b (Hib)
- Pneumococcal
- Polio
- Influenza
- Measles, mumps, and rubella (MMR)
- Varicella (chickenpox)
- Hepatitis A
- Meningococcus
- Human papillomavirus (a.k.a. HPV)

Affix a copy of your official immunizations/vaccination record on this page.

VACCINATIONS – QUICK REFERENCE

Vaccine Name	Date Administered	Physician	Any side effects noted?

VITAL SIGNS/PHYSICAL EXAMS – At-A-Glance

Keep track of this information after your annual physicals/doctor's visits to help monitor your health from year to year.
(For *Heart* and *Lungs* indicate whether exams were normal or irregularities were noted by your doctor.)

Date M/D/Y	Blood Pressure	Choleste-rol Total	HDL Choles.	LDL Choles.	Triglyce-rides	Heart	Lungs

VITAL SIGNS/PHYSICAL EXAMS – At-A-Glance (cont'd)

Date M/D/Y	Blood Pressure	Choleste-rol Total	HDL Choles.	LDL Choles.	Triglyce-rides	Heart	Lungs

VITAL SIGNS/PHYSICAL EXAMS – At-A-Glance (cont'd)

Date M/D/Y	Blood Pressure	Choleste-rol Total	HDL Choles.	LDL Choles.	Triglyce-rides	Heart	Lungs

GENDER-SPECIFIC & OTHER EXAM RESULTS

Note the results of routine tests such as PSA/prostate, blood glucose, Pap/HPV, thyroid function, colonoscopy, etc.

Exam Name	______________________________	
Test Date	**Results**	**Physician/Lab Site/Notes**
/ /		
/ /		
/ /		
/ /		
/ /		
/ /		

Exam Name	______________________________	
Test Date	**Results**	**Physician/Lab Site/Notes**
/ /		
/ /		
/ /		
/ /		
/ /		

GENDER-SPECIFIC & OTHER EXAM RESULTS (cont'd)

Exam Name	____________________	
Test Date	Results	Physician/Lab Site/Notes
/ /		
/ /		
/ /		
/ /		
/ /		
/ /		

Exam Name	____________________	
Test Date	Results	Physician/Lab Site/Notes
/ /		
/ /		
/ /		
/ /		
/ /		
/ /		

GENDER-SPECIFIC & OTHER EXAM RESULTS (cont'd)

Exam Name	___________________________	
Test Date	**Results**	**Physician/Lab Site/Notes**
/ /		
/ /		
/ /		
/ /		
/ /		
/ /		

Exam Name	___________________________	
Test Date	**Results**	**Physician/Lab Site/Notes**
/ /		
/ /		
/ /		
/ /		
/ /		
/ /		

GENDER-SPECIFIC & OTHER EXAM RESULTS (cont'd)

Exam Name	______________________	
Test Date	Results	Physician/Lab Site/Notes
/ /		
/ /		
/ /		
/ /		
/ /		
/ /		

Exam Name	______________________	
Test Date	Results	Physician/Lab Site/Notes
/ /		
/ /		
/ /		
/ /		
/ /		
/ /		

GENDER-SPECIFIC & OTHER EXAM RESULTS (cont'd)

Exam Name	____________________	
Test Date	Results	Physician/Lab Site/Notes
/ /		
/ /		
/ /		
/ /		
/ /		
/ /		

Exam Name	____________________	
Test Date	Results	Physician/Lab Site/Notes
/ /		
/ /		
/ /		
/ /		
/ /		
/ /		

GENDER-SPECIFIC & OTHER EXAM RESULTS (cont'd)

Exam Name	______________________________	
Test Date	**Results**	**Physician/Lab Site/Notes**
/ /		
/ /		
/ /		
/ /		
/ /		
/ /		

Exam Name	______________________________	
Test Date	**Results**	**Physician/Lab Site/Notes**
/ /		
/ /		
/ /		
/ /		
/ /		
/ /		

IMAGING & RADIOLOGY TESTS

MRIs, CAT scans, ultrasound/sonograms, mammograms, PET scans, X-rays, etc. Suggestion: Make a habit of getting a printed copy of the results/findings of these tests for your personal files.

Date	Test Name	Where taken?	Results
Where kept: *Indicate where you keep your copy of the digital images or films and the findings report*			
Where kept:			
Where kept:			
Where kept:			
Where kept:			

IMAGING & RADIOLOGY TESTS (cont'd)

Date	Test Name	Where taken?	Results
Where kept:			
Where kept:			
Where kept:			
Where kept:			
Where kept:			

IMAGING & RADIOLOGY TESTS (cont'd)

Date	Test Name	Where taken?	Results
Where kept:			
Where kept:			
Where kept:			
Where kept:			
Where kept:			

IMAGING & RADIOLOGY TESTS (cont'd)

Date	Test Name	Where taken?	Results
Where kept:			
Where kept:			
Where kept:			
Where kept:			
Where kept:			

IMAGING & RADIOLOGY TESTS (cont'd)

Date	Test Name	Where taken?	Results
Where kept:			
Where kept:			
Where kept:			
Where kept:			
Where kept:			

IMAGING & RADIOLOGY TESTS (cont'd)

Date	Test Name	Where taken?	Results
Where kept:			
Where kept:			
Where kept:			
Where kept:			
Where kept:			

IMAGING & RADIOLOGY TESTS (cont'd)

Date	Test Name	Where taken?	Results
Where kept:			
Where kept:			
Where kept:			
Where kept:			
Where kept:			

DISEASES, CHRONIC ILLNESSES & CONDITIONS
(other than allergies)

Date Diagnosed	Diseases, Chronic Illnesses, Conditions

DISEASES, CHRONIC ILLNESSES & CONDITIONS
(other than allergies)

Date Diagnosed	Diseases, Chronic Illnesses, Conditions

Important information regarding specific illnesses:

Condition:	
Name(s) of doctors(s) used:	
Course of treatment/ Prescriptions:	
Hospitalizations/ Surgeries:	**Y / N** *(if Y, elaborate)*
Outcome/Issue Resolved?	

Condition:	
Name(s) of doctors(s) used:	
Course of treatment/ Prescriptions:	
Hospitalizations/ Surgeries:	**Y / N** *(if Y, elaborate)*
Outcome/Issue Resolved?	

Important information regarding specific illnesses (cont'd):

Condition:	
Name(s) of doctors(s) used:	
Course of treatment/ Prescriptions:	
Hospitalizations/ Surgeries:	**Y / N** *(if Y, elaborate)*
Outcome/Issue Resolved?	

Condition:	
Name(s) of doctors(s) used:	
Course of treatment/ Prescriptions:	
Hospitalizations/ Surgeries:	**Y / N** *(if Y, elaborate)*
Outcome/Issue Resolved?	

Important information regarding specific illnesses (cont'd):

Condition:	
Name(s) of doctors(s) used:	
Course of treatment/ Prescriptions:	
Hospitalizations/ Surgeries:	**Y / N** *(if Y, elaborate)*
Outcome/Issue Resolved?	

Condition:	
Name(s) of doctors(s) used:	
Course of treatment/ Prescriptions:	
Hospitalizations/ Surgeries:	**Y / N** *(if Y, elaborate)*
Outcome/Issue Resolved?	

NOTES/EXTRA INFORMATION
Re: My Medical History

8 HOSPITALIZATIONS & SURGERIES

HOSPITALIZATIONS & SURGERIES

Date:
Hospital Name & Location:

Length of stay:
Reason:

Surgery? Y / N
Type of surgery, if applicable:

****

Date:
Hospital Name & Location:

Length of stay:
Reason:

Surgery? Y / N
Type of surgery, if applicable:

****

Date:
Hospital Name & Location:

Length of stay:
Reason:

Surgery? Y / N
Type of surgery, if applicable:

****

HOSPITALIZATIONS & SURGERIES (cont'd)

Date:
Hospital Name & Location:

Length of stay:
Reason:

Surgery? Y / N
Type of surgery, if applicable:

****

Date:
Hospital Name & Location:

Length of stay:
Reason:

Surgery? Y / N
Type of surgery, if applicable:

****

Date:
Hospital Name & Location:

Length of stay:
Reason:

Surgery? Y / N
Type of surgery, if applicable:

****

HOSPITALIZATIONS & SURGERIES (cont'd)

Date:
Hospital Name & Location:

Length of stay:
Reason:

Surgery? Y / N
Type of surgery, if applicable:

****

Date:
Hospital Name & Location:

Length of stay:
Reason:

Surgery? Y / N
Type of surgery/doctor name:

****

Date:
Hospital Name & Location:

Length of stay:
Reason:

Surgery? Y / N
Type of surgery, if applicable:

****

HOSPITALIZATIONS & SURGERIES (cont'd)

Date:
Hospital Name & Location:

Length of stay:
Reason:

Surgery? Y / N
Type of surgery, if applicable:

****

Date:
Hospital Name & Location:

Length of stay:
Reason:

Surgery? Y / N
Type of surgery, if applicable:

****

Date:
Hospital Name & Location:

Length of stay:
Reason:

Surgery? Y / N
Type of surgery, if applicable:

****

HOSPITALIZATIONS & SURGERIES (cont'd)

Date:
Hospital Name & Location:

Length of stay:
Reason:

Surgery? Y / N
Type of surgery, if applicable:

****

Date:
Hospital Name & Location:

Length of stay:
Reason:

Surgery? Y / N
Type of surgery, if applicable:

****

Date:
Hospital Name & Location:

Length of stay:
Reason:

Surgery? Y / N
Type of surgery, if applicable:

****

HOSPITALIZATIONS & SURGERIES (cont'd)

Date:
Hospital Name & Location:

Length of stay:
Reason:

Surgery? Y / N
Type of surgery, if applicable:

****

Date:
Hospital Name & Location:

Length of stay:
Reason:

Surgery? Y / N
Type of surgery, if applicable:

****

Date:
Hospital Name & Location:

Length of stay:
Reason:

Surgery? Y / N
Type of surgery, if applicable:

****

NOTES/EXTRA INFORMATION
Re: Hospitalization & Surgeries

9 DOCTORS

APPOINTMENTS WITH DOCTORS

Date	Doctor	Reason for Visit/Outcome

APPOINTMENTS WITH DOCTORS (cont'd)

Date	Doctor	Reason for Visit/Outcome

APPOINTMENTS WITH DOCTORS (cont'd)

Date	Doctor	Reason for Visit/Outcome

APPOINTMENTS WITH DOCTORS (cont'd)

Date	Doctor	Reason for Visit/Outcome

APPOINTMENTS WITH DOCTORS (cont'd)

Date	Doctor	Reason for Visit/Outcome

APPOINTMENTS WITH DOCTORS (cont'd)

Date	Doctor	Reason for Visit/Outcome

APPOINTMENTS WITH DOCTORS (cont'd)

Date	Doctor	Reason for Visit/Outcome

APPOINTMENTS WITH DOCTORS (cont'd)

Date	Doctor	Reason for Visit/Outcome

MY DOCTORS: CONTACT INFORMATION

You can tape your doctor's business card in this space or just write in your doctor's full name and contact info. Include address, phone/fax #s & email. Also note your PCP. If former doctor information is kept in this book, make sure to indicate in some way which doctors you no longer see.

Dates Used--

From:

To:

Conditions Treated:

Dates Used--

From:

To:

Conditions Treated:

Dates Used--

From:

To:

Conditions Treated:

MY DOCTORS: CONTACT INFORMATION (cont'd)

Dates Used--

From:

To:

Conditions Treated:

Dates Used--

From:

To:

Conditions Treated:

Dates Used--

From:

To:

Conditions Treated:

MY DOCTORS: CONTACT INFORMATION (cont'd)

Tape your doctors' business cards
in these spaces or write in contact info.

Dates Used--
From:

To:

Conditions
Treated:

Dates Used--
From:

To:

Conditions
Treated:

Dates Used--
From:

To:

Conditions
Treated:

MY DOCTORS: CONTACT INFORMATION (cont'd)

Dates Used--

From:

To:

Conditions Treated:

Dates Used--

From:

To:

Conditions Treated:

Dates Used--

From:

To:

Conditions Treated:

MY DOCTORS: CONTACT INFORMATION (cont'd)

Tape your doctors' business cards
in these spaces or write in contact info.

Dates Used--

From:

To:

Conditions Treated:

Dates Used--

From:

To:

Conditions Treated:

Dates Used--

From:

To:

Conditions Treated:

MY DOCTORS: CONTACT INFORMATION (cont'd)

Dates Used--
From:

To:

Conditions Treated:

Dates Used--
From:

To:

Conditions Treated:

Dates Used--
From:

To:

Conditions Treated:

MY DOCTORS: CONTACT INFORMATION (cont'd)

Tape your doctors business cards
in these spaces or write in contact info.

Dates Used--
From:

To:

Conditions
Treated:

Dates Used--
From:

To:

Conditions
Treated:

Dates Used--
From:

To:

Conditions
Treated:

MY DOCTORS: CONTACT INFORMATION (cont'd)

Dates Used--
From:

To:

Conditions
Treated:

Dates Used--
From:

To:

Conditions
Treated:

Dates Used--
From:

To:

Conditions
Treated:

NOTES/EXTRA INFORMATION
Re: My Doctors

10 PRESCRIPTIONS

PREFERRED PHARMACIES
(in order of preference/use)

Pharmacy Name:

Address (incl. zip code):

Telephone #:

Is a particular pharmacist at this location familiar with you and your prescriptions? Yes____ No____

If Yes, Pharmacist's Name ______________________________

****

Pharmacy Name:

Address (incl. zip code):

Telephone #:

Is a particular pharmacist at this location familiar with you and your prescriptions? Yes____ No____

If Yes, Pharmacist's Name ______________________________

****

Pharmacy Name:

Address (incl. zip code):

Telephone #:

Is a particular pharmacist at this location familiar with you and your prescriptions? Yes____ No____

If Yes, Pharmacist's Name ______________________________

****

PRESCRIPTIONS

Running list of prescriptions received (filled & unfilled)

Date Received	Drug Name/ Condition Treated *(if applicable, include dates taken)*	Prescribing Doctor	Filled? Y or N

PRESCRIPTIONS (cont'd)

Running list of prescriptions received (filled & unfilled)

Date Received	Drug Name/ Condition Treated *(if applicable, include dates taken)*	Prescribing Doctor	Filled? Y or N

PRESCRIPTIONS (cont'd)

Running list of prescriptions received (filled & unfilled)

Date Received	Drug Name/ Condition Treated *(if applicable, include dates taken)*	Prescribing Doctor	Filled? Y or N

PRESCRIPTIONS (cont'd)

Running list of prescriptions received (filled & unfilled)

Date Received	**Drug Name/ Condition Treated** ***(if applicable, include dates taken)***	**Prescribing Doctor**	**Filled? Y or N**

PRESCRIPTIONS (cont'd)

Running list of prescriptions received (filled & unfilled)

Date Received	Drug Name/ Condition Treated *(if applicable, include dates taken)*	Prescribing Doctor	Filled? Y or N

PRESCRIPTIONS (cont'd)

Running list of prescriptions received (filled & unfilled)

Date Received	Drug Name/ Condition Treated *(if applicable, include dates taken)*	Prescribing Doctor	Filled? Y or N

PRESCRIPTIONS (cont'd)

Running list of prescriptions received (filled & unfilled)

Date Received	Drug Name/ Condition Treated *(if applicable, include dates taken)*	Prescribing Doctor	Filled? Y or N

PRESCRIPTIONS (cont'd)

Running list of prescriptions received (filled & unfilled)

Date Received	Drug Name/ Condition Treated *(if applicable, include dates taken)*	Prescribing Doctor	Filled? Y or N

PRESCRIPTIONS -- LABELS

Affix the prescription labels from your pharmacy receipts on these pages to keep a record of dosages & regimens (It may be helpful to write the name of the condition the drug was treating above the label for easy reference.)

Example:
Pneumonia

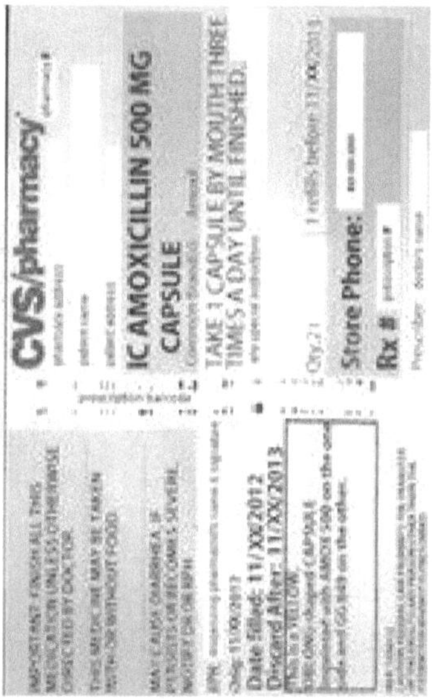

PRESCRIPTIONS -- LABELS

PRESCRIPTIONS -- LABELS

PRESCRIPTIONS -- LABELS

PRESCRIPTIONS -- LABELS

PRESCRIPTIONS -- LABELS

PRESCRIPTIONS – LABELS

PRESCRIPTIONS – LABELS

PRESCRIPTIONS – LABELS

PRESCRIPTIONS – LABELS

11 OTC DRUGS & SUPPLEMENTS

OVER-THE-COUNTER DRUG & SUPPLEMENT USE

List any OTC drugs and supplements/vitamins that you are taking for the first time or those that you take repeatedly. Mention these to your doctor before getting new prescriptions and/or before surgery to avoid potential interactions & complications.

Date(s) Taken	Brand Name/ Generic Name	WhyTaken?	Dosage

OVER-THE-COUNTER DRUG & SUPPLEMENT USE (cont'd)

Date(s) Taken	Brand Name/ Generic Name	Why Taken?	Dosage

OVER-THE-COUNTER DRUG & SUPPLEMENT USE (cont'd)

Date(s) Taken	Brand Name/ Generic Name	Why Taken?	Dosage

OVER-THE-COUNTER DRUG & SUPPLEMENT USE (cont'd)

Date(s) Taken	Brand Name/ Generic Name	Why Taken?	Dosage

NOTES

NOTES

NOTES

NOTES

Made in United States
Troutdale, OR
11/03/2026

56847379R00070